Generis
PUBLISHING

Managing of Sports and Determining the Difference Between the Chronological and Biological Age

Josip Miočić

Title: **Managing of Sports and Determining the Difference Between the Chronological and Biological Age**

ISBN: 979-8-89966-489-2

Author: Josip Miočić

Cover image: www.pixabay.com

Publisher: Generis Publishing
Online orders: www.generis-publishing.com
Contact email: info@generis-publishing.com

CONTENTS

Managing Multiple Sclerosis (MS): The Impact of exercise on adaptive aapacities in recreational athletes diagnosed with Multiple Sclerosis

assoc. prof . Josip Miočić, PhD – Centre for Physical Activity and Student Sport, University of Zadar

Milica Komšo, MD – General Hospital Zadar

Assoc. Prof. Tonći Jerak, PhD – Centre for Physical Activity and Student Sport, University of Zadar

Abstract: Multiple sclerosis (MS) is a chronic neurodegenerative disease characterized by highly variable symptoms that may fluctuate within a single day. Individuals diagnosed with MS experience changes in both functional and cognitive capacities, necessitating continuous adjustments in lifestyle and physical activity. Within a fitness context, the use of resistance bands and training aids such as stationary bicycles or ergometers enables safe, adapted exercise on days when symptoms are stable. However, the primary goal of physical activity in the context of MS is to establish a sustainable form of movement that remains feasible even in the presence of symptoms. This research applied inferential statistical analysis using Spearman's rank-order correlation to assess the relationships between variables, resulting in a correlation matrix with Spearman's rho values and corresponding p-values. Findings indicate positive effects of regular physical activity in mitigating MS symptoms such as fatigue, mobility difficulties, and cognitive impairments. Beyond physical benefits, exercise contributes to a greater sense of control over the disease and enhances social and emotional well-being.

A specific feature of this study is its focus on individuals living on the Dalmatian coast, where climatic factors—especially elevated temperatures for most of the year—further influence exercise adaptations, particularly due to the common occurrence of heat intolerance in people with MS. Accordingly, the importance of a personalized exercise approach is emphasized, aligned with current recommendations from the National MS Society (USA), which include physical activity guidelines tailored to all levels of functional ability.

Keywords: multiple sclerosis, exercise intervention, Spearman's correlation, recreational sport.

INTRODUCTION

When a person—including a recreational athlete—is diagnosed with a condition such as multiple sclerosis (MS), understanding the role of physical activity in disease management becomes crucial. Studies have shown that regular exercise can positively impact various aspects of life for individuals with MS, including mood enhancement, improved strength, balance, and functional mobility, as well as reduced fatigue (Latimer-Cheung et al., 2013). Although physical inactivity and sedentary behavior are relatively common among people with MS, growing evidence supports the idea that individualized exercise can improve both physical and psychological health and quality of life (Latimer-Cheung et al., 2013; Motl & Pilutti, 2012). Nevertheless, challenges such as fatigue, heat intolerance, and mobility limitations often hinder consistent exercise participation, especially in recreational athletes. These symptoms require specific modifications to exercise routines (Motl & Pilutti, 2012). Consequently, fitness routines must evolve to reflect the fluctuating symptoms of MS in recreational athletes. This approach aligns with current guidelines emphasizing individualized exercise programming to optimize benefits and minimize risks (Dalgas et al., 2019). While recreational athletes may not maintain previous fitness levels, they continue to adapt their routines to incorporate exercise as an integral part of daily life (Androja et al., 2020). Ongoing adaptation and mindful engagement with one's capabilities and limitations are key to successful long-term disease management through physical activity (Miočić & Komšo, 2020). This study addresses the lack of understanding regarding how recreational athletes with MS adapt their training regimens over time in response to evolving symptoms, particularly from the perspective of lived experience (Du et al., 2024). There is a recognized need to explore subjective experiences of exercise among individuals with MS to inform realistic, sustainable, and motivating exercise programs that account for the challenges of this unpredictable disease. The aim of this paper is to explore and present the personal experience of exercise adaptation in recreational athletes living with MS and to compare these insights with current scientific knowledge. The study combines personal narrative and literature review to highlight the importance of a flexible, individualized approach to physical activity in MS. Research questions include: How do recreational athletes with MS perceive and adapt their training over time?, How can these subjective experiences be reconciled with scientific recommendations for physical activity?, What are the most common challenges to maintaining regular training among individuals with MS?

Context and Personal Perspective

For many individuals, physical exercise was an integral part of their identity and daily routine prior to being diagnosed with multiple sclerosis (MS). As long-time recreational athletes, they were accustomed to a dynamic lifestyle that included various forms of physical activity such as hiking, water sports, running, functional training, and occasional participation in amateur competitions. However, the diagnosis of MS introduced a profound shift in how these individuals perceive, experience, and engage in physical activity. The onset of initial symptoms—such as chronic fatigue, heat sensitivity, and intermittent limb weakness—significantly affected their ability to maintain previous levels of physical performance. Initially, many continued with their usual training intensity, often ignoring the changes. However, as Motl and Pilutti (2012) point out, individuals with MS who do not adjust their activity intensity may experience worsening symptoms and further declines in quality of life.

Moving forward, recreational athletes are compelled to adopt a different mindset—transitioning from someone who "pushes physical limits through training" to someone who exercises with the goals of preserving functionality, reducing symptoms, and maintaining mental stability and social inclusion. As such, training becomes perceived less as a means to athletic progression and more as a therapeutic tool. This shift in perspective is supported by existing literature, which recognizes physical activity as an "informal intervention for symptom management, preserving independence, and improving quality of life in individuals with MS" (Latimer-Cheung et al., 2013, p. 1801). This process necessitates acceptance of flexibility in training—adapting the duration, intensity, and type of activity to the body's daily condition (Miočić et al., 2020). According to Rodríguez and colleagues (2021), on days when symptoms are mild, individuals engage in short functional workouts using body weight, whereas during periods of pronounced fatigue, exercise routines consist of light stretching and breathing exercises. This approach aligns with the recommendations of Dalgas et al. (2019), who emphasize the importance of individualized and appropriate physical activity in people with MS. Beyond physical benefits, exercise helps individuals retain a sense of continuity and control—maintaining connection with the "athlete I was before the diagnosis" (Miočić & Komšo, 2020). As Grazioli et al. (2019) suggest, although the athletic identity is altered, it remains present—now redefined as that of a person who consciously engages in exercise as a form of self-care and self-sustenance.

METHODS

This study employed a mixed methods design, integrating qualitative autoethnographic approaches with quantitative descriptive statistics. This combination enabled the integration of the subjective dimension of personal experience with objective patterns of behavior and perception within a broader population of individuals diagnosed with multiple sclerosis (MS) who engage in physical activity.

Qualitative Component. The qualitative portion of the study was based on autoethnography, a research method that blends autobiographical writing with ethnographic analysis (Ellis, Adams, & Bochner, 2011; Sparkes, 2000). Participants—recreational athletes diagnosed with MS—maintained diary entries, retrospective notes, and reflective essays over a six-month period. The collected narrative data covered topics such as training adaptations, emotional responses, and shifts in perceptions of physical activity. The data were analyzed using the thematic analysis method proposed by Braun and Clarke (2006), which allows for the identification of patterns of meaning within qualitative data. Three key themes emerged from the analysis: Redefinition of athletic identity, Flexibility and adaptation of the training process, Psychological significance and function of exercise in managing disease symptoms.

Quantitative Component. The quantitative segment of the research involved descriptive statistical analysis derived from a structured online questionnaire. The study sample included 40 recreational athletes with MS, aged 28 to 62 years ($M = 44.2$; $SD = 8.1$), consisting of 60% women ($n = 24$) and 40% men ($n = 16$). The questionnaire comprised the following thematic sections:Demographic data (age, gender, disease duration), Exercise habits (frequency, duration, type of activity), Perceived exercise intensity (self-assessed), and Self-assessment of the impact of MS symptoms on daily functioning and ability to engage in physical activity.

The goal of the quantitative analysis was to identify patterns in exercise behavior and perception among individuals with MS, and to compare these findings with the results of the qualitative (autoethnographic) analysis, in order to construct a more comprehensive understanding of the experience of physical activity in the context of MS.

For additional scientific rigor, an inferential statistical method was applied—Spearman's rank-order correlation (Field, 2013)—to examine the relationships among four variables: disease duration, exercise frequency, exercise intensity, and the perceived impact of MS symptoms. The resulting data analysis yielded a correlation matrix with Spearman's rho values and associated p-values for significance testing.

RESULTS AND DISCUSSION

The quantitative findings serve to complement the qualitative insights, affirming that the author's personal experiences are not isolated, but rather reflect broader patterns among recreational athletes with multiple sclerosis (MS) who strive to maintain an active lifestyle. Both qualitative and quantitative analyses reveal a complex and dynamic adaptation process in physical activity among individuals with MS, with a particular emphasis on the importance of maintaining a sense of identity and control through movement.

Practical Implications of the Research Findings

The study results suggest several key guidelines for working with recreational athletes diagnosed with MS, especially those with a history of regular training:

- A) Flexibility in Training Program Design Training programs should be dynamic and adaptable to the individual's current physical condition. This involves modifications in intensity, duration, and type of activity according to daily fluctuations in symptoms (Dalgas et al., 2019).

- B) Preservation of Identity Through Movemen. For recreational athletes, exercise is not merely a physical activity, but part of their personal identity. Training should support a sense of continuity with their "athletic self," even if through modified forms of physical activity.

- C) Psychosocial Support Through Exercis. Survey results show that 92.5% of participants report a positive psychological effect of exercise. Incorporating physical activity as a therapeutic tool within multidisciplinary rehabilitation can play a key role in preserving mental health.

- D) Interdisciplinary Collaboratio. Optimal support for individuals with MS involves collaboration among professionals such as physiotherapists, kinesiologists, neurologists, and psychologists, ensuring that physical activity is integrated into holistic health care.

Key Descriptive Statistics 85% of participants ($n = 34$) reported the need to modify their training regimen after MS diagnosis. 72.5% ($n = 29$) exercised 2–4 times per week, while only 10% ($n = 4$) trained more than four times weekly. The most common types of activity reported were: Walking (78%), Stretching (62%), Swimming (38%), Light functional training (35%) and 47.5% identified fatigue as the greatest barrier to regular training, followed by balance and coordination difficulties (25%).

A significant 92.5% (n = 37) of participants stated that engaging in physical activity positively affected their mental health, particularly in relation to stress, anxiety, social connectedness, and perceived control.

Further Interpretation and Thematic Findings Redefinition of Athletic Identity.

1. Autoethnographic reflections revealed a gradual, emotionally demanding shift in identity—from someone who trains to increase fitness and performance to someone who exercises for self-preservation. This transformation is supported by the survey results, where 92.5% reported that exercise contributes to maintaining psychological stability. This aligns with previous research highlighting the mental health benefits of physical activity in individuals with MS (Latimer-Cheung et al., 2013).
2. Adaptation of the Training Process. Descriptive statistics showed that the majority (85%) regularly adjust the form, duration, and intensity of their exercise based on daily symptom variability. As previously noted, the most common activities include walking (78%), stretching (62%), swimming (38%), and functional training (35%). These activities are typically low to moderate in intensity, consistent with current recommendations for people with MS (Dalgas et al., 2019). The author's personal experience further validates the necessity for flexibility, as days with more pronounced symptoms often limit activity to light stretching and breathing exercises.

Table 1. Most Common Types of Activity Among Recreational Athletes with MS

Type of Activity	Percentage (%)
Walking	78%
Stretching	62%
Swimming	38%
Functional training	35%

3. **Perceived Barriers and the Importance of Adaptation.** Fatigue was identified as the main barrier to physical activity by 47.5% of participants, while 25% reported balance-related problems. These findings align with the literature, which identifies fatigue as one of the strongest predictors of reduced physical activity in people with MS (Motl & Pilutti, 2012). Despite these challenges, most participants found ways

to maintain some form of physical activity, shifting exercise from a "recreational" practice to a means of **self-care**, as evidenced by the survey results. This redefinition of the role of physical activity in participants' lives highlights the importance of **developing individualized and flexible training programs** that account for the physical, emotional, and identity-related dimensions of living with this chronic condition.

Table 2. Perceived Main Barriers to Engaging in Physical Activity

Type of Barrier	**Percentage (%)**
Fatigue	47.5%
Balance problems	25%
Other barriers	27.5%

Study Limitations, Like any research, this study has certain limitations: **Sample size**: The quantitative analysis is based on a relatively small sample (n = 40), limiting generalizability. **Subjectivity of the autoethnographic approach**: While autoethnography provides rich, in-depth insights, it is inherently subjective and cannot represent all individuals with MS. **Self-reported data**: All quantitative data rely on self-reporting, which may be subject to social desirability bias and inaccurate assessments. **Symptom variability in MS**: Due to the heterogeneous nature of the disease, drawing universal conclusions applicable to all individuals with MS is challenging.

Table 3. Frequency of Physical Activity in Recreational Athletes with MS

Exercise Frequency	**Percentage (%)**
2–4 times per week	72.5%
More than 4 times per week	10%
Less than 2 times per week	17.5%

Correlational Analysis. Spearman's rank correlation analysis was conducted to examine relationships among four variables: duration of illness, frequency of exercise, intensity of exercise, and perceived impact of MS symptoms. The results (Pallant, 2020) show that none of the correlations reached statistical significance (all $p > 0.05$). However, a slight positive relationship was observed between exercise frequency and exercise intensity ($\rho = 0.260$), as well as between exercise frequency and perceived symptom impact ($\rho = 0.265$). Correlations involving illness duration were weak or negligible.

Table 4. Spearman's Correlation Between Key Variables

Variables	ρ (rho)	p-value
Duration of illness – Exercise frequency	–0.017	0.919
Duration of illness – Exercise intensity	0.088	0.593
Duration of illness – Symptom impact	0.116	0.481
Exercise frequency – Exercise intensity	0.260	0.110
Exercise frequency – Symptom impact	0.265	0.103
Exercise intensity – Symptom impact	0.151	0.360

CONCLUSION

This study highlights that, despite the numerous challenges brought on by a diagnosis of multiple sclerosis (MS), physical activity remains a crucial factor in preserving quality of life, personal identity, social inclusion, and psychological stability among recreational athletes. By integrating autoethnographic insight with quantitative data, it was found that individuals with MS rarely abandon exercise altogether. Instead, they redefine and adapt it, using training as a **therapeutic tool**. The findings point to several key needs: A sensitized, multidimensional approach by professionals who understand the specific challenges of living with MS, The development of adaptable training models, offering flexibility according to fluctuating symptoms, Greater awareness of the psychological value of exercise, even when performed in minimal amounts. To deepen the analytical scope of the study, a Spearman's rank-order correlation was conducted, revealing a slight positive association between exercise frequency and intensity ($\rho = 0.26$), and between exercise frequency and perceived symptom impact ($\rho = 0.265$). Ultimately, physical activity emerges as **a** space of resistance against the disease—a domain where the individual retains an active role in their own health, not only through bodily movement but also through the meaning they assign to motion, rhythm, and the discipline of everyday social life. Future research could expand on this work by: Conducting longitudinal studies tracking changes in exercise engagement across different stages of the disease, Comparing distinct subgroups (e.g., previously active vs. inactive individuals with MS), Including larger and more diverse samples, as well as in-depth qualitative interviews to better understand individual adaptation strategies and Exploring the potential of digital tools and online exercise programs for people with MS — particularly in the context of accessibility and self-monitoring of progress.

REFERENCES

1. Androja, L., Miočić, J., Bilić, Ž., & Komšo, M. (2021). Frequency of peripheral nerve injuries in athletes of certain sports clubs in the city of Zadar. *Acta Kinesiologica, 15*(1), 127–132. https://doi.org/10.51371/issn.1840-2976.2021.15.1.1
2. Braun, V., & Clarke, V. (2006). Using thematic analysis in psychology. *Qualitative Research in Psychology, 3*(2), 77–101. https://doi.org/10.1191/1478088706qp063oa
3. Dalgas, U., Langeskov-Christensen, M., Stenager, E., & Riemenschneider, M. (2019). Exercise as medicine in multiple sclerosis—Time for a paradigm shift: Preventive, symptomatic, and disease-modifying aspects and perspectives. *Current Neurology and Neuroscience Reports, 19*(11), 88. https://doi.org/10.1007/s11910-019-1004-7
4. Du, L., Xi, H., Zhang, S., Zhou, Y., Tao, X., Lv, Y., Hou, X., & Yu, L. (2024). Effects of exercise in people with multiple sclerosis: A systematic review and meta-analysis. *Frontiers in Public Health, 12*, Article 1387658. https://doi.org/10.3389/fpubh.2024.1387658
5. Ellis, C., Adams, T. E., & Bochner, A. P. (2011). Autoethnography: An overview. *Forum: Qualitative Social Research, 12*(1), Article 10. https://doi.org/10.17169/fqs-12.1.1589
6. Field, A. (2013). *Discovering statistics using IBM SPSS statistics* (4th ed.). Sage Publications.
7. Grazioli, E., Tranchita, E., Borriello, G., Cerulli, C., Minganti, C., & Parisi, A. (2019). The effects of concurrent resistance and aerobic exercise training on functional status in patients with multiple sclerosis. *Current Sports Medicine Reports, 18*(12), 452–457. https://doi.org/10.1249/JSR.0000000000000661
8. Latimer-Cheung, A. E., Pilutti, L. A., Hicks, A. L., Ginis, K. A. M., Fenuta, A. M., MacKibbon, K. A., & Motl, R. W. (2013). Effects of exercise training on fitness, mobility, fatigue, and health-related quality of life among adults with multiple sclerosis: A systematic review to inform guideline development. *Archives of Physical Medicine and Rehabilitation, 94*(9), 1800–1828.e3. https://doi.org/10.1016/j.apmr.2013.04.020
9. Mitchell, C. H., Brushant, T. M., Shivani, A., Belzberg, A. J., Corrino, J. A., & Fayad, L. M. (2014). MRI of sports-related peripheral nerve injuries. *AJR American Journal of Roentgenology, 203*(5), 1075–1084. https://doi.org/10.2214/AJR.13.11844

10. Miočić, J., & Komšo, M. (2020). Važnost tjelesnog vježbanja za osobe s dijagnosticiranom multiplom sklerozom. *Zbornik Sveučilišta Libertas, 5*(5), 27–34. https://doi.org/10.46672/zsl.5.5.2

11. Miočić, J., Androja, L., & Čular, D. (2020). Understanding the significance of cannabidiols and their possible use in sport. *International Journal of Innovative Science and Research Technology, 5*(7). [ISSN: 2456-2165]

12. Motl, R. W., & Pilutti, L. A. (2012). The benefits of exercise training in multiple sclerosis. *Nature Reviews Neurology, 8*(9), 487–497. https://doi.org/10.1038/nrneurol.2012.136

13. Pallant, J. (2020). *SPSS survival manual: A step-by-step guide to data analysis using IBM SPSS* (7th ed.). McGraw-Hill Education.

14. Rodríguez Fuentes, G., Silveira Pereira, L., Ferradáns Rodríguez, P., & Campo Prieto, P. (2022). Therapeutic effects of the Pilates method in patients with multiple sclerosis: A systematic review. *Journal of Clinical Medicine, 11*(3), 683. https://doi.org/10.3390/jcm11030683

15. Sparkes, A. C. (2000). Autoethnography and narratives of self: Reflections on criteria in action. *Sociology of Sport Journal, 17*(1), 21–43. https://doi.org/10.1123/ssj.17.1.21

FEATURES OF PLAYING ESPORTS GAMES AND THE IMPACT ON STATUS OF STUDENTS AND ATHLETES

Josip Miočić
University College Aspira
Molatska ulica 11 a, 23000 Zadar, Hrvatska
+00385 996895762
josip.miocic@szgz.hr

Luka Androja
University College Aspira
Domovinskog rata 65, 21000 Split, Hrvatska
+00385 996895762
luka.androja@aspira.hr

Original scientific paper

Abstract: Esports represents the playing of organized and competitive video game play at the amateur and professional level, where it is associated with large financial rewards and earnings. In the modern world, it is a form of sport or entertainment, which attracts a large number of spectators and participants, who are involved online or at large competitions, the possibility of watching "live" in sports arenas is provided. The competitions take place in the form of leagues and tournaments, they are sponsored, and the prize fund is growing every day and in the modern world it competes with the most popular traditional sports. Given that this is a relative novelty for the Croatian sports and social market, the purpose of this research is to analyze some features of esports in order to see and recognize its status and impact on the student and sports population. This paper aims to determine the relationship between the variables that are considered important for shaping esports and its impact on the student and sports population. Knowledge of esports was highlighted through general questions and through regression analysis of some features of esports.

Keywords: esports, regression analysis, features,

JEL Classification: O14, Z29

1. Introduction

In the modern world we live in, digitization and new e-technologies have brought significant and accelerated changes in human life. Digitization is a new reality and a reality in all segments of society (Androja, Miočić & Zdrilić, 2021). In everyday life, including in the life of athletes, the word "digitalization" appears more and more often (Miočić, Androja & Bilić, 2020). Work, everyday life and communication have taken on a completely different form, where the changes are dynamic and radical, and have been reflected in sports by the development of new opportunities for entertainment and recreation, as well as new competitive sports. One of the most popular and fastest growing, especially in developed economies, is esports. Esport as a term derives and comes from the already existing concept of traditional sports. Sport in human culture has developed into more than a mere recreational content and now receives a predominantly competitive content caused by economic progress. As early as the ancient Olympic Games, there was a certain professionalization of sports, and it referred to people, i.e. athletes, who had certain predispositions for it. Sport today exists in two dimensions, one is of a recreational nature, while the other has a professional dimension, which implies that a person lives on the income he earns from playing a certain sport. How much and how and in which social population esports is developing in Croatia is the research question of this work.

The purpose of this research is to look at sport in its basic dimensions and influences, such as knowledge of the rules of the game, as well as the conditions and the way it develops in Croatia. For research and evaluation of the level of development, specific variables were set that lead to answers related to the level of development of esports in Croatia in the researched population. Therefore, variable research was set as the goal of esports and esports player research, namely: participants, free time, financial resources, equipment availability and access. The research hypothesis, as well as the expected results, are set as a claim that the degree of development, as well as the development of esports in Croatia, is at a lower level among the researched population compared to other developed countries.

2. Esports

With the development of civilization, competitive sports appeared as one of its products, which went from rough and vulgar games without special rules to civilized modern sports (Elias & Dunning, 1986). As a rule, sport has a competitive character and connects the audience, fans and spectators. With regard to the mentioned basic features of sports, esports within the framework of e-technology meets all the features of traditional sports disciplines, as well as their competitive character. Due to the popularity of modern technologies and video games among the younger population, competitions have developed in which many players want to measure and compare their abilities with other players. As a product of the above, there are organizations that have developed competitive systems to enable these players to compete (Jonasson & Thiborg, 2010). Competitive esports are based on player activities on a specific interface with the help of digital technology. Sports competitions in esports take place in defined leagues and tournaments, and professional teams or individual players participate in them. In the last decade, esports is one of the fastest growing entertainment industries with high audience growth (Anušić, 2020). The development of e-sports in Croatia lags behind modern advanced societies, although progress is visible, so today there are two large regional sports leagues in Croatia, namely the A1 Adria League and the Esports B League, which are currently the top competitions in which you can play more widely Croatian environment. A tournament called Dota Pit is held every year, while the big Dota 2 tournament is also the most popular esports tournament in Croatia. The main significance of the Dota Pit tournament is the popularization of the sport in the Croatian sports IT community.

There are currently around 385 million people watching esports (online or in stadiums) worldwide, and this is predicted to grow to 589 (Polman et al., 2018). Examples of this type of game are DOTA 2 and League of Legends. The question arises of shaping the characteristics of esports players. Since esports does not contain traditional elements of physical training and activity, there is still the problem of defining competitive video game playing as a sport (Laakkonen, 2014). The same problem of defining sport is also related to some other interesting sports games, such as chess or darts, which can be played today, and are played in the "e" form. Although playing video games is incomparable to traditional sports in terms of physical fatigue per unit of time, it is still not true that there is no physical investment that an esports player must make to be a professional (Anušić, 2020). The main characteristic of esports, and of esports players during playing and training, is long-term sitting, as well as the efforts that the body and brain endure from hours of standing in an upright position of the spine and arms. It is also important to point out that long-term looking at the monitor can result in vision damage, as well as electromagnetic radiation that can damage the player's health. This creates a need for organized occupational therapists, teams and trainers who take care of their fitness. Therefore, it follows that esports is conceived in a similar way to well-known traditional sports. Just like in traditional sports where there are followers of handball, football, volleyball, water polo, skiing, cycling, etc., so in esports there are followers related to game titles, such as "League of Legends", "DOTA2", "CSGO" etc. (Leoonard, 2008).

Each of these titles usually has its own loyal audience that follows the events within just one title. One of the esports genres is completely based on traditional sports. Considering the complexity of esports and its connection with traditional sports, it is more appropriate to define esports according to what esports does and how the expressive feature of this new concept will be found. The most important feature of esports is that we have opposing competitive players. The outcome and result of their game is completely determined in the virtual world for which electronic equipment is used. In esports, the main element of the game is the interaction of players who give commands through an electronic interface, so the result is achieved in virtual space. Viewers of esports content, unlike traditional sports, are closely tied to the use of computers and streaming services while watching esports content. In some countries, such as South Korea, television channels are dedicated to the daily broadcast of esports content. In Europe, this trend is less accepted. Most viewers watch esports content through popular streaming providers, including Twitch, Youtube, and Chinese streaming services Douyu and Huya (Popper, 2014). During the end of the season and the final professional tournaments at the regional and world level, spaces and halls and stadiums decorated and adapted for sports are activated. They are physically filled with esports audiences. In traditional sports, depending on the sport and the audience, it is a regular practice for the audience from a particular city to cheer on their sports team in a weekly competition at the stadium where the sports competition is held. A very similar feature is present in Esports. This feature is very important because it includes additional services, such as catering and hotel and other services, which achieve significant economic profit.

3. Development of esports and similarities and differences with traditional sports

Esport was created in 1999, although the term itself was mentioned earlier. The first tournaments and competitions took place over a LAN connection in the 70s and 80s of the last century in high schools and universities. In the beginning, competitions were held by playing against computers, or bots created by video game manufacturers. In 1980, the World Championship for Space Invaders was held. However, esports became what it is when the Counter-Strike World Championship was broadcast and distributed. By allowing public viewing, they sent the gaming event to interested viewers, and since then the pressure on competitors and organizers has increased. Since then, competitions from almost every multiplayer video game have been held regularly, with the inevitable growth of prize pools awarded to participants and winners of esports competitions. Esports as a new sports industry does not function without a foundation (Brodie, 2017), which is the video game industry. Where there has been a demand for a competitive scene where players can test their talents and the need to compete (Draven, 2020). With the development of digital technology, the first tournaments and competitions appeared almost parallel to the first video games, although professional esports players are mentioned several decades later (Tl.net, 2011). Every year, esports breaks previously set records, and the space for growth remains stable and connected to new generations growing up in a fully digitalized world. The first appearance of the sport can be traced back to the creation of the first video games, such as Pong or Spacewars (Tl.net, 2011).

In the United Kingdom at Oxford University in 1972, the first tournament was Spacewar with a prize in the form of a 28-year subscription to the globally popular Rolling Stone magazine (Farockmanesh, 2012). The organizing committee of the 2024 Paris Olympics has been in talks with the International Olympic Committee (IOC) and various professional sports organizations to consider the possibility of including sports in the Olympic Games programme. Considering the interest of the audience and the changes that are present in the globalized world, it is definitely time to expand the concept of sport and its definition. Expanding the sport by accepting a new sport would make the Olympics more interesting and acceptable to the younger generation. The President of the IOC, Mr. X. Bach stated that there are two difficulties in presenting sport as an Olympic event. In his opinion, this requires a higher degree of restriction of violent types of games, but also the adoption of a global sports regulatory body (Associated Press, 2017. With the development and availability of broadband Internet, more and more users have access to higher Internet speeds, which allows them to play more demanding games online with others players in real time (Edge, 2013). Therefore, internet speed is a key factor in the development of video games and ultimately esports in modern society.

Eathlete? The characteristics of an esports athlete differ from a traditional athlete. The traditional concept of an athlete is related to the perception of a well-prepared athlete with a muscular body. However, this is not what characterizes esports players. The claim says that both need training, strategy, teamwork, good reflexes and perseverance (LeClaire, 2007). Like traditional athletes, esports take part in the training process with the help of professional teams, coaches and specialized staff for each competition. Therefore, the question arises, what are the basic sports characteristics of an athlete? Also, accordingly, the question arises, is esports a sport or is it entertainment and lucrative income of the modern age? The biggest difference between sports and traditional sports is physical activity, i.e. movement, but also physical and psychophysical readiness and stability. Claims say that there is almost no physical activity in esports, but this is not true (TL.net. 2022). It is necessary to convince the general public that it makes sense to broadcast a specialized television program that would broadcast exclusively sports. So, the path to acceptance of sport as a new sport takes place through the Internet and TV industry. Given the available data in the literature and the high amounts of financial resources involved in esports, how is it possible that despite the large amount of money, esports still has strong opponents (Electronic Arts Reports Q2 FY20 Financial Results, 2020). One of the causes is according to the available literature, the scandals that happened in esports related to doping state that professional esports players presented information about doping in the form of "adderall". Along with doping, there have been suspicions of "the use of illegal technology. Illegal technologies include the use of "Hacks" (commonly called cheating in games) to create "Aimbots" (a computer-controlled character that mimics a player, a term sometimes used for people who cheat - use of Aimbot and/or Wallhack) giving an unfair advantage to the players who use them (Hore, 2020). Therefore, anomalies present in all types of sports are reflected in the domain of undesirable situations and unsportsmanlike behavior in esports. Experts in the literature state that esports is a good combination stimulating online games and physically exhausting sports and that this is exactly what meets the needs of the coming modern generations.

4. Who can be an e-sports player?

On general, anyone can participate in esports segments, but not everyone can become a professional esports player. Being good at the game is only part of the necessary abilities and skills and predispositions that make up the connections and abilities that will help you climb the competitive ladder.

No, what limits can an individual player go and what psychomotor abilities should he possess, is the question we are dealing with today. Observing the anthropological status of an individual, certain dimensions develop under the influence of external social and other factors of growth and development. Reflexes, reactions, cognitive dimensions, perception, speed, precision, rhythmic coordination, etc. are essential for successful esports players. Also, we must not ignore the conative dimensions (personality traits) which, as in classic sports, make a big difference between athletes, and also among esports players (Brodie, 2017).

5. Research part

The research is a product of the authors' previous studies on the subject, in which, alongside the analysis and examination of the global esports scene, special attention was also given to the domestic esports scene. Many international organizations are built upon the quality and success of Croatian esports players (such as “Perkz”); however, unfortunately, there is still no developed esports team in Croatia capable of competing on the global stage with larger organizations (Wolf, 2019). Esports in Croatia is still far from being fully recognized and accepted as such. The study also analyzed and presented the level of usage and interest in esports among members of 12 sports clubs and the student population in the area of the City of Zadar.

5.1. Subject and goal of the research

The subject of the research is to present some features and meanings of regression analysis for esports segments. The hypothesis of the research is the assertion that the degree of development, as well as the development of esports in Croatia, i.e. in the city of Zadar, is at a lower level among the researched population compared to other more economically developed countries. Also, explore the possibilities of its application in terms of playing sports video games within esports. The purpose of the questionnaire is to determine the level of consumption of esports among members of sports clubs and students in the city of Zadar.

6.2. Methods, variables and sample of respondents

Data collection was carried out on the basis of a proportional stratified sample, since it belongs to the category of random samples and enables the assessment of the degree of reliability of the conclusions about the examined parameters. The research was conducted through a questionnaire through several basic questions in order to obtain an overview of the sample taken through basic statistical parameters. After conducting the survey questionnaire on the basic questions, the second part of the survey was conducted, which refers to certain specifics important for playing video games (availability of IT and electronic equipment, free time and financial resources).

Also, the regression results are presented as an example of the importance of the respondent's status following the previous variables and guided by the main criterion variable. All questions were analyzed. The aim of this work is to determine the relationship between variables, that is, to determine statistical dependencies and indicators. The regression analysis technique was used to determine the strength of dependence of individual variables because it is based on a regression model that analytically expresses and shows the connection of phenomena. The research is a product of previous research, and the sample is represented by members of sports clubs (26 coaches, athletes and sports workers) and 72 students of the University of Zadar (N=49). More men (92%) than women (8%) participated in the research. Those aged 20 to 22 prevail (85% of respondents)

7. Results and discussion

The main part of the research relates to general questions and was conducted through a survey. The first question was to determine how many respondents play any of the esports games. The answer was that as many as 88.6% of respondents play an esports game. The second question was about the interest in playing traditional sports and playing esports. 65.5% of respondents are more interested in playing sports, whether recreational, amateur or professional, while 34.5% of respondents say that playing esports is more interesting to them.

Then, the next question related to the respondents' knowledge of the concept of sport, and the answer was mostly: "I know completely", which leads to the conclusion that the respondents are sufficiently familiar with the aforementioned. It is also visible in table 1 - "How familiar are you with the term "esports"?"). The largest number, 72% of respondents believe that they are: "completely familiar", followed by 13% that they are "partially familiar". While a significantly smaller percentage of respondents, 6%, consider that they are "neither familiar nor unknown", 7% of respondents consider that they are "partially unfamiliar", and only 2% of respondents consider that they are "not fully familiar".

Table 1. *Results of the question - How familiar are you with the term „esports"?*

Completely not familiar	Partially not familiar	Neither familiar nor nonfamiliar	Partially familiar	Completely familiar
2%	7%	6%	13%	72%

Then, there was the question that referred to the period of playing video games within the esports (Only for respondents who play esport). The answer (Table 2) showed us that respondents are playing esport for 3-5 years (84%), then some of them play more than 5 years (12%) and some of them play up to 2 years (6%).

Table 2. *Results of the question - How long have you been playing video games within esports?*

Up to 2 years	3 – 5 years	More than 5 years
6%	84%	12%

7.1. Data processing

The second part of the research is related to multivariate data analysis - regression analysis. The results of the research show the criteria for evaluating the impact on playing video games: availability of electronic equipment, free time, financial resources explain 68.7% of the variance in the overall comprehensibility of sports evaluation criteria (*R2 = 0.687, F (89) = 29.156, p = 0.000*). Furthermore, the availability of electronic equipment (*β = 0.078, t = 0.901 & p = 0.000*) and financial resources (*β = 0.352, t = 3.412 & p = 0.000*) are shown to be significant positive predictors of overall comprehensibility, while leisure time (*β = 0.382, t =2.576 & p = 0.370*) doesn't show significant contribution (Table 3).

Table 3. *Regression analysis of the influence of individual elements as a predictor of the overall impact on playing video games*

	B (*Unstandardized coefficient)*	**Beta** *(Standardized coefficient)*	**t**	**Sig.**
Availability of IT - electronic equipment	0.094	0.078	0.901	**0.000**
Leisure time	0.037	0.382	2.576	0.370
Financial resources	0.037	0.352	3.412	**0.000**

The importance of "availability of IT and electronic equipment" could be argued as a key factor for starting sports activities through the type of set criteria. Also, it's not just any kind of electronic equipment. Electronic equipment must fall under high and modern technology in order to follow the trends.Due to constant updates, the system requires frequent software and especially hardware upgrades. Every year eigre companies present new eigres and their new requirements according to market monitoring. For example, playing eigare through the prism of fun at home will be easily implemented through minimal requirements, while for more serious gaming it is necessary to have hardware compatible with the maximum requirements of the game. If a player plays video games with minimum requirements, it is unlikely that they will succeed in the world of esports, because they will not be able to keep up with all the upcoming titles and upgrades of the existing ones.

Also, playing on minimum requirements often brings a slower reaction in the game itself, not because of the "inability" of the player, but because of lagging (popularly known as lag in gaming). Players mostly complain about lower FPS (frame per second) due to worse graphics cards and processors. Newer eigers require more gigabytes on the graphics cards themselves, and cannot be upgraded like motherboards, but a completely new graphics card must be purchased. In this way, a player can lose matches due to older electronic equipment. "Financial resources" are consistent with the variable described above. Buying new electronic equipment meets the requirements of the games that the player plays. A certain budget is required. A player must constantly invest in equipment if he wants to progress. The players are predominantly a younger population, as we can see from the example of this paper that 85% of respondents are aged 20-22. This population does not have enough financial resources for constant technical

Table 4. *Regression analysis – Respondents' work status and participation in esports*

	B *(Unstandardized coefficient)*	**Beta** *(Standardized coefficient)*	**t**	**Sig.**
Student	1.75	0.264	3.100	**0.003**
Professionally employed in the association	0.149	0.256	3.200	**0.002**
The athlete who has status in the association	1.840	0.360	3.836	**0.000**
An amateur athlete	0.292	-0.134	-1.255	0.213
Unemployed status	0.156	0.311	3.593	**0.001**
Part-time athlete	-0.132	0.119	1.105	0.273
Part-time sports employee	0.012	0.126	1.853	0.068

The significance of the "student" variable is expected because they are the ones most involved in playing any type of video game. New generations were brought up with modern technologies, so they are an unavoidable dimension of everyday life. The general results of the survey were presented, which show that they are more in favor of classic sports, but the positive influence of video games has certainly been proven through various studies. Research has shown that eigre contributes to the development of logical thinking, problem-solving skills and the improvement of critical thinking. Children also develop better hand-eye coordination and precision. E-games can greatly help in improving reading, language learning and arithmetic (Brčić, 2020). The relationship between the question about the frequency of playing and the question about the assessment of their own mental and physical abilities shows that all the examined students, no matter how often they play, rate their abilities better than average. There are no relationships that would indicate significant differences in the abilities of those who play and those who do not (Haramija, Njavro and Vranešić, 2020). "Professionally employed in the association" and "Athlete who has a status in the association" contribute to the importance of the regression analysis. Since it is a relatively young population as a sample of respondents, and according to the general survey, it can be concluded that the respondents often play eigre in their free time. We often witness advertisements on the covers of various video games, such as FIFA 21, FIFA 22, NBA 2K22, etc. The advertisements mostly feature young professional athletes who mostly play e-games in their free time. They have the main influence on the rest of the population. Since athletes have a lot of free time during the break from training, it is assumed that they spend a lot of time playing e-games in their free time, according to the survey and other claims. According to the sample of respondents, the "unemployed status" is also shared by the younger population, who spend most of their free time playing e-games.

8. Conclusion

Esports represent a potential flywheel of our society in the field of sports, entertainment and economy. The aim of the work was to determine the relationship between the variables that are considered important for the structure of esports, which represents new concepts in our social environment in the prism of competitive play, but also of free time. Traditional sports are increasingly competing with e-sports on a global level through organized competitions in the form of tournaments or leagues. In Croatian esports, to understand the current situation, this research tried to bring esports closer to society (users) and potential users. Based on the conducted research and the results of the survey questionnaire filled out by the members of the sports associations and the student population from the city of Zadar, several topics were opened up inspired by the questions from the constructed survey questionnaire. The research substantiated the questions and established the fact that a large number of respondents know the concept of esports and that they have been playing video games for several years, primarily in their free time. The population that plays and understands esports are students, among whom the majority are athletes and the unemployed. Also, the results show that esports on the Croatian market is in its infancy and is gradually developing. There is significant potential for its spread in society through the target population of users in the future.

9. References

Androja, L., Miočić, J. & Zdrilić, I. (2021) Basic characteristics and significance of factor analysis in the process of digitalization of football clubs in the city of Zadar. Interdisciplinary Management Research XVII.

Anušić, V. (2020): *Esport-nova grana industrije zabave* (Master thesis)

Associated Press. (2017). "Paris Olympic bid committee is open to esports on 2024 Olympic program".ESPN. Available at: http://www.espn.co.uk/olympics/story/_/id/20286757/parisopen-esports-competition-2024-summer-olympics (October 28th 2021)

Brčić, I. (2020). Utjecaj video igara na djecu. In medias res, 9 (17), 2669-2684. https://doi.org/10.46640/imr.9.17.6

Brodie, C. (2017) This technology is boosting literacy rates in India and beyond. Digitalempowers.com. Available at: https://digitalempowers.com/technology-boosting-literacy-rates-india-beyond/ (October 28th 2021)

Draven, D. (2020) 10 Reasons Why The O.G. GameBoy Was So Successful. Thegamer.com. Available at: https://www.thegamer.com/original-gameboy-succsess/ (October 28th 2021)

Edge, N. (2013) Evoltuion of the Gaming Experience: Live Video Streaming and the Emergence of a New Web Community. Inquiriesjournal.com. Available at: http://www.inquiriesjournal.com/articles/821/evolution-of-thegaming-experience-live-video-streaming-and-the-emergence-of-a-new-web-community (October 28th 2021)

Electronic Arts Reports Q2 FY20 Financial Results (2020). Ir.ea.com. Available at: https://ir.ea.com/pressreleases/press-release-details/2019/Electronic-Arts-Reports-Q2-FY20-Financial-Results/default.aspx (October 28th 2021)

Farokmanesh, M (2012): First game tournament 'Intergalacitc Spacewars Olympics', held 40 years ago, polygon.com. Available at: https://www.polygon.com/2012/10/20/3529662/first-game-tournamentintergalactic-spacewar-olympics-held-40-years (October 28th 2021)

Haramija, P., Njavro, Đ. i Vranešić, P. (2020). Videoigre i njihov utjecaj na uspjeh, sposobnosti i svjetonazor studenata. Obnovljeni Život, 75. (1.), 93-108. https://doi.org/10.31337/oz.75.1.7

Hore J. (2020): Who is Dr DisRespect? Net value, settings, and more, theloadout.com. Available at: Who is Dr Disrespect? Net worth, settings, and more | The Loadout (October 28th 2021)

Jonasson, K., & Thiborg, J. (2010). Electronic sport and its impact on future sport. Sport in Society, 13, 287 - 299.

Jurko, D., Čular, D., Badrić, M. & Sporiš, G. (2015) Osnove kineziologije. Zagreb: sportska-knjiga

LeClaire Jennifer (2007): 'World of Warcraft ' Wows 8 million subscribers, Ecommercertimes.com. Available at: https://www.ecommercetimes.com/story/55135.html (October 28th 2021)

Leoonard, D. (2008): Calling master chief, money.cnn.com. Available at: https://money.cnn.com/2008/08/05/technology/mlg.fortune/index.htm?postversion=2008082113 (October 28th 2021)

Miočić, J., Androja, L. & Bilić, Ž. (2020) The impact of the covid-19 pandemic on the psychosomatic status of athletes and sports stakeholders. International journal of advanced research (Indore), 8 (10), 412-417 doi:10.21474/IJAR01/11672.

Polman, R., Trotter, M., Poulus, D., & Borkoles, E. (2018). eSport: Friend or Foe? In Joint International Conference on Serious Games (pp. 3-8). Springer, Cham

Popper B. (2014): Justin.tv the live video pioneer that that birthed Twitch, officially shuts down, Theverge.com. Available at: https://www.theverge.com/2014/8/5/5971939/justin-tv-the-live-videopioneer-that-birthed-twitch-officially-shuts (October 28th 2021)

Sarkar, Samit (January 12, 2018). „MLS launching esports league for FIFA 18 World Cup“. Polygon. MLS launching esports league for FIFA 18 World Cup - Polygon (October 28th 2021)

Tl.net (2011): eSports: A Short History of Nearly Everything. Available at: https://tl.net/forum/starcraft-2/249860-esports-a-short-history-of-nearly-everything (October 28th 2021)

Wolf. J (2019): Sources: Huni agrees to two-year, $2.3 million extension with Dignitas, espn.com. Available at: https://www.espn.com/esports/story/_/id/28059409/sources-huni-agrees-two-year-23-million-extension-dignitas (October 28th 2021)

WOMEN'S FOOTBALL PROSPECTS IN CITY OF ZADAR AND ZADAR COUNTY

research article

doc. dr.sc. Josip Miočić, Športska zajednica Grada Zadra,
josip.miocic@szgz.hr

Abstract: The research conducted is focused on status and prospects of women's football in the city of Zadar and Zadar County. Since football is the most famous sport in the world, and thus also in the mentioned area, it transcends the category of sport. The concept of sport is not unambiguous and it has no unique generally accepted definition. The aim of the research was to determine the satisfaction of the respondents with the status and popularity of women's football in the city of Zadar and Zadar County.The research used a method of survey and a suitable questionnaire in order to investigate satisfaction of respondents with social status of women's football in the city of Zadar and Zadar County. The respondents included 78 sports employees, coaches and players of women's football from the city of Zadar and Zadar County area. The aim of this research is to establish the level of satisfaction of the respondents with social status of women's football and the level of its popularity growth in the city of Zadar and Zadar County. Moreover, the aim is also to establish the level of socialization of such population achieved by participating in women's football. According to this research it is possible to confirm the hypothesis that participants are not completely satisfied with social status and the popularity growth of women's football in the city of Zadar and Zadar County and that the level of socialization is improved by participating in such activity.

Key words: football, women, prospects, satisfaction, social status

Introduction

As numbers show, football is one of the most popular sports in the world and as such, in Croatia. Its popularity is defined and enabled by the possibility of participation for both male and female sportspeople (Grgić, 2018). According to the Croatian Football Association (HNS) data there are 124.064 registered football players while there are about 22 million in the world. Women's football in Croatia is insufficiently represented since there are 1264 registered female football players which is only 1%

of overall number of registered football players (HNS, 2019). Thus, football is still considered as men's sport in Croatian society which is obvious because of: the amount of funds invested, the number of active players, clubs, leagues, media interest, number of stadiums, etc. (Softić, 2018). At the same time, women's football as such is still not properly developed because of the problem of gender stereotypes in our society. In their research with respondents from student population, Bosnar and Žugaj concluded that even educated population sees football as primarily men's sport (Bosnar, Žugaj 2009). However, "women's football is a sport in the world of women's sports that transcends the area of sports and becomes a serious dispute in many international councils and governing bodies" (FIFA, 2019). As confirmed in the last FIFA Women's World Cup in Lyon, France 2019, most of women's sports in the world are in the shadow of men's. However, football, as the most important of the less important things in the world, provides a chance to establish itself and achieve the "importance", i.e. equality. Of course, women's football is primarily a sport and secondarily a tool for achieving certain goals. So, terms "women and men" should not be taken for granted since in its core it is a game played by women and men. Thus, it is obvious that women's football is not sufficiently represented and recognized in the city of Zadar and Zadar County and as such is "fighting" for its existence. Thomas Bach, the president of IOC[1], is promoting and insisting on principles of gender equality in Olympic Movement project and he also promotes proper terminology in football. Hence, there are questions: Are there prospects in women's football? Can women's football be just football and not a tool for fighting inequality? Are there ways to promote women's football and what are they?

Football and sport

Sport is a matter of interest for different profile of scientists, sociologists, medics, economists, communicologists, etc. in modern society. Since the concept of sport is not unambiguous and it has no unique generally accepted definition, the paper states social component accepted by most sociologists that we "should ask what activities are defined as sport and why in a certain society" (Coakley, 2007). As a social institution, sport depends to a large extent on dominant culture, i.e. values and norms of a society it belongs to which is of great importance considering the context of this paper. According to the Sports Act in Croatia, sport is defined as "any physical and psychological activity that person does according to a set of rules, with aim to compete with an opponent or an opponent's team by applying a set system of scoring that defines a winner" (Sports Act). Sport is a part of social needs of all individuals, a universal mean of understanding and cooperation among people with aim of physical and

[1] International Olympic Committee

spiritual upbringing, vitality and health, social relations and attitudes, defence readiness and quality of life, and it also represents the category of economy.

Today's football represents, without doubt, the most popular sport in Croatia and it has features of acyclic activity. It belongs to a dynamic group of sports in which two teams, 11 players each, compete against each other, establish the ball flow and try to achieve a score during the match. Stamina, speed, strength, coordination, accuracy and flexibility form the hierarchy of motor abilities (Dujmović, 2006). Even though football can be marked as "male" sport, there is a positive social attitude towards women's participation. Leskovar (2012) identified positive attitude towards women's football on a sample of both male and female students of high school. Rural areas in our country and Zadar County represent the most conservative parts of society. If a positive attitude towards women's football exists in such areas, we can conclude that it is time for institutions to do their part in order to develop it. Thus, the aim of this research is to establish the attitude towards women's football in rural area on a sample of people of different gender and age.

Women in footbal

Equality in football should be one of the basic goals of contemporary sports, as set and conducted by FIFA. Since different efforts to promote equality are introduced by society, governing bodies, etc., prejudices have reduced in everyday life and in football, but they still exist. Thus, traditional values which consider football as an area dominated by masculine values are beginning to decrease (Coakley, 2007). According to Talleu, in a handbook "Gender equality in sports: access for girls and women to sport practices", it is still necessary to make an effort to achieve gender equality in football because there is still great unused potential in society. Sport can give positive contribution to society: doing sports promotes mutual respect, resourcefulness and understanding by connecting people of different gender, race, religion, age and economical background. Sports activities, if managed well, can be tools for fighting discrimination, prejudices and stereotypes (Talleu, 2011). One can question the state of women's football in countries where national teams did not qualify for world championships and in that way did not enter the international scene. Insufficiently developed sports infrastructure and insufficient funds as well as overall support is generally a serious problem of women's team sports in Croatia and especially football which position is considered as insufficiently recognised. However, women's football has recently achieved some progress in Croatia. Researches and strategies such as "Together for the future of football" from 2019 to 2024, Bosnar Kovačević in 2011, Herman in 2016, Medo in 2018, etc. all show a certain progress that also includes investment in infrastructure, competition system, coach education, number of clubs and, most importantly, the number of new young sportswomen. 1937, when the first women's football club "Bata" in Borovo was formed, is considered as the beginning of official women's football. Whereas today, according to HNS data, "from total of 118 316 registered players of football and futsal in Croatia, only 2106 are female, including younger age groups" which is worrying. But these data and the following should be taken with precaution because in last few years there has been an improvement in this area (Baršić, 2018). There are 1 732 football clubs registered in Croatian Football Association with only 38 women's clubs. Among judges, there are 2239 men and only 19 women (HNS, 2013). Such status can be explained in several ways: insufficient care, not enough interest within sports institutions responsible for development of football, gender stereotypes in society, negligence and resistance of overall society regarding this matter. Stereotypes possibly influence parents when choosing sports for girls and there is still a very conservative attitude regarding the choice of sports for girls, like for example: volleyball, basketball, swimming, etc. Gregurić research from 2018 is based on social aspect of sex and gender and it confirmed that gender stereotypes can inhibit the development of women's football as well as all gender stereotypical activities. (Gregurić, 2018).

Women football in Croatia

It should be stressed that since 2012 there has been a continuing growth of registered female players of football which is a result of various factors and processes done by public administration and overall society. "There are five centres of women's football in Croatia (Zagreb, Varaždin, Split, Osijek, Rijeka) which are equivalent to men's football" and they organise camps where educated coaches work with girls and promote football (HNS, 2019). This presents infrastructural grounds for development of women's football. It is obvious that the existence of such centres helps to form a system of competitions, women's sports clubs, quality matches and educated staff which is a key moment for further development of women's football. Currently, in Croatian official system of competitions, women's clubs compete in 1st HNLŽ (Croatian Football League for Women) and 2nd HNLŽ and in regional system of competing for youth. This trend is marked by achieved sports results of clubs as well as national teams on international competitions (participating in qualifications for Euro League - ŽNK Split, etc.), professionalization of players' status, possible creation and participation of Croatian clubs in regional league with aim of raising the quality. Countries which have well developed women's football (Austria, Hungary, Slovakia, etc.) and which have market interest would participate in the competition.

In the last few years there has been a vivid continuing growth of women's football in the city of Zadar and Zadar County. There has been an increase in number of active clubs (3 clubs) as well as the number of girls and women (around 190) who play football. This means that they are becoming increasingly important factor of women's football in this area. Along with volleyball, swimming, rhythmic gymnastics, basketball and several individual sports, women's football makes up a sum of sports which dominates in popularity in the city of Zadar and Zadar County (ŠZGZ, 2019). Considering social context, presence and role of modern technologies in lives of youth, all should be used to promote football.

Methods

In order to investigate the satisfaction of respondents with social status of women's football in the city of Zadar and Zadar County, method of survey was used and appropriate questionnaire was formed. The survey represents a quantitative form of research and it gathered data about different attitudes and opinions (satisfaction) of respondents which identified possible changes needed in order to improve social status of women's football. The questionnaire included four areas of research: social status of women's football in the city of Zadar and Zadar County, popularity of women's football in the city of Zadar and Zadar County, quality of women's football and women's football.

Respondents

The sample of respondents includes 78 sports employees, coaches and female players of women's football in the city of Zadar and Zadar County. Respondents actively participate in women's football and they are representative sample for this area of research. Total number includes 6 coaches, 3 presidents and secretaries of clubs and the rest (69) are players of Women's football club Donat, Futsal super Chiks and Football club Abeceda sporta. This paper analyses results of the questionnaire which was answered by 78 respondents, i.e. those who were training at the moment of research. Respondents filled in the questionnaire after training in appropriate facility. The questionnaire was first tested on a sample of 5 respondents and later was given to the other participants in this research. All profiles of respondents were included (coaches, players and sports employees). It consists of 11 questions organised in two parts: general and research. First part is related to general data, while the other part consists of questions which have the aim to answer suggested hypotheses of this paper. After conducting this survey, questionnaires in printed form were imported in a program LimeSurvey and then exported in specialized SPSS data analysing program.

Aims

The aim of this paper is to establish the satisfaction of respondents with social status of women's football in the city of Zadar and Zadar County as well as the level of popularity growth of women's football and also to directly identify the level of socialization of such population achieved by playing women's football. In accordance with the aim, it is possible to generate hypothesis that participants are not satisfied with the status of women's football in the city of Zadar and Zadar County and that the level of socialization is improved because of their participation in women's football.

Results

After the survey was conducted, respondents' answers were analysed. Results showed that there were more female respondents (75%) than men (25%) and majority of respondents (80%) were those aged between 15 and 20. A group of questions related to the satisfaction with social status of women's football in the city of Zadar and Zadar County crystallised the answer that social status is unsatisfactory as seen in answers to the question (Table 1) *How satisfied are you with social status of women's football in the city of Zadar and Zadar County?* The majority of respondents (80%) are completely dissatisfied with the status of women's football, while 8 % are partly dissatisfied. Fewer respondents (9.4%) answered that they are neither satisfied nor dissatisfied. 2.6% respondents are partly satisfied; however no one is completely satisfied.

Table 1: *Question results - How satisfied are you with social status of women's football in the city of Zadar and Zadar County?*

Completely dissatisfied	Partly dissatisfied	Neither satisfied nor dissatisfied	Partly satisfied	Completely satisfied
80%	8%	9.4%	2.6%	-

There was a clear answer concerning growth and popularity of women's football (table 2) where 63% respondents answered the popularity is growing (as expected concerning the profile of respondents), 26,66% answered it neither grows nor it does not grow and 12,04% answered it does not grow.

Table 2: *Question results – Does popularity of women's football in the city of Zadar and Zadar County grow?*

It does not grow	Neither grows nor it does not grow	It grows
12,04%	26,66%	61,3%

Question *Does women's football have lower quality than men's football*? generated similar percentage of answers; 21,33% answered yes, neither yes nor no was answered by 33,33%, while 45,33% answered no.

Table 3: *Question results – Does women's football have lower quality than men's football?*

No	Neither yes nor no	Yes
45,33%	33,33%	21,33%

Question *Does participation in women's football influence your inclusion in society?* generated answers as follows: yes in 60%, neither no nor yes in 25,34% and no in 14,66%.

Table 4: *Question results – Does participation in women's football influence your inclusion in society?*

No	Neither no nor yes	Yes
14,66%	25,34%	60%

Good response from respondents is due to wish and motivation of sports employees, coaches and players of women's football to improve and open new prospects for women's football. This research and its results gained from 78 respondents opened new topics, questions that are necessary to deal with in the future: is women's football a tool for fighting for women's rights and appreciation of women's football in rural areas of referred county; since contemporary football is business, how fit is women's football for such aspect considering market interest in Croatia? This research and its results which included 78 respondents opened several other topics that need to be discussed in the future.

Conclusion

Women's football in the world is far more developed than in Croatia, including the city of Zadar and Zadar County. As established by the results of this research, the reason is not only the negative attitude of the general population towards women's football, but also insufficient effort in the development of women's football by institutions. In order to follow the models of more developed countries in this area, especially in Europe, in the city of Zadar and Zadar County, the guidelines and goals of FIFA for the development of women's football should be adhered to.These include: improving the infrastructure needed for women's football, increasing the number of members in the football school, increasing the number of women's competitions, enrolling women in technical and management areas of football such as refereeing, training and administration, organizing seminars for coaches, referees and analyzing and monitoring women's technical development. football. With all of the above in mind, it is important to stress that infrastructure is also essential for men's football. Improving the conditions for women's football can gain prospects in men's football as well. This research found that respondents are not satisfied with the status and popularity of women's football in the city of Zadar and Zadar County and its quality. It has also been confirmed that playing football helps female footballers to integrate into societies of events. Moreover, women's football should not only be a tool for gender equality, but it is an exciting sport, perhaps currently less attractive than men's, but with perspectives and new ideas of improvement it can develop into a sport that can satisfy society in general in the same way as men football.

References

1. Baršić, M. (2018). Žene i nogomet u hrvatskom društvu: što futsal ima s tim? (Doctoral dissertation, University of Zagreb. Faculty of Kinesiology. Department of Kinesiological Anthropology and Methodology. Chair of Kinesiological Psychology, Sociology and Methodology.). Žene i nogomet u hrvatskom društvu: što futsal ima s tim? | Repository of Faculty of Kinesiology, University of Zagreb (unizg.hr)
2. Bosnar K. and Žugaj, S. (2009). Gender typing of sports in Croatian university students. In. Doupona Topič, M. And Ličen, S. (Eds.): Sport, culture & society: an account of views and perspectives on social issues in a continent (and beyond), Ljubljana: University of Ljubljana, Faculty of Sport:161-164. Bosnar K. and Žugaj, S. (2009). Gender typing of sports in Croatian university students. In. Doupona Topič, M. And Ličen, S. (Eds.): Sport, culture & society: an account of views and perspectives on social issues in a continent (and beyond), Ljubljana: University of Ljubljana, Faculty of Sport:161-164. - Google pretraživanje
3. Coakley J. (2007). Sports in Society: Issues and Controversies. New York: McGraw-Hill Sports in Society: Issues and Controversies (mheducation.com)
4. Dujmović, P. (2006). Škola suvremenog nogometa. Zagreb: Zagrebački nogometni savez. (Book) https://bib.irb.hr/datoteka/954262.RAZVOJ_NOGOMETAA.pdf
5. Gregurić, M. (2018). Spol i rod: sociološka analiza hrvatskog ženskog nogometa (Doctoral dissertation, University of Zagreb. Faculty of Kinesiology. Department of Kinesiological Anthropology and Methodology. Chair of Kinesiological Psychology, Sociology and Methodology.). 198148143.pdf (core.ac.uk)

6. Grgić, S. (2018). A Brief History of Women's Football in Croatia/Yugoslavia during the Interwar Period. Časopis za suvremenu povijest, 50(3), 557-580. A Brief History of Women's Football in Croatia/Yugoslavia during the Interwar Period (srce.hr)

7. Hrvatski nogometni savez (2019) Službene web stranice. Skinuto s mreže 03.09.2019. s adrese: https://hns-cff.hr/

8. Leskovar, S. (2012). Stav prema ženskom nogometu kod srednjoškolaca (diplomski rad). Zagreb: Kineziološki fakultet Sveučilišta u Zagrebu 67-Kovacevic.indd (hrks.hr)

9. Fédération Internationale de Football Association (2019) Službene web stranice. Skinuto s mreže 03.09.2919. s adrese: https://www.fifa.com/womens-football/

10. Talleu C. (2011). Ravnopravnost spolova u športu: dostupnost športskih aktivnosti djevojčicama i ženama. Priručnici o dobroj praksi, br. 2. Vlada RH, Ured za ravnopravnost spolova, Zagreb. Ured za ravnopravnost spolova - Priručnik o dobroj praksi Vijeća Europe „Ravnopravnost spolova u športu – Dostupnost športskih aktivnosti djevojčicama i ženama" (gov.hr)

11. Softić, J. (2018). Nogomet u Istarskoj županiji (University of Pula. Faculty of Educational Sciences.). Nogomet u Istarskoj županiji | Digitalni repozitorij Sveučilišta Jurja Dobrile u Puli (unipu.hr)

12. Zakon o sportu. Narodne novine, br. 71/06, 150/08, 124/10, 124/11, 86/12, 94/13, 85/15, 96/16. Zakon o sportu - Zakon.hr

13. Kosinac, Z. (2002). Kineziterapija sustava za kretanje, Split: Sveučilište u Splitu, 78-80. 2.

14. Findak, V. (1999). Metodika tjelesne i zdravstvene kulture, Zagreb: Školska knjiga, 222.

Managing Multiple Sclerosis (MS): The Impact of exercise on adaptive aapacities in recreational athletes diagnosed with Multiple Sclerosis

assoc. prof . Josip Miočić, PhD – Centre for Physical Activity and Student Sport, University of Zadar

Milica Komšo, MD – General Hospital Zadar

Abstract: Multiple sclerosis (MS) is a chronic neurodegenerative disease characterized by highly variable symptoms that may fluctuate within a single day. Individuals diagnosed with MS experience changes in both functional and cognitive capacities, necessitating continuous adjustments in lifestyle and physical activity. Within a fitness context, the use of resistance bands and training aids such as stationary bicycles or ergometers enables safe, adapted exercise on days when symptoms are stable. However, the primary goal of physical activity in the context of MS is to establish a sustainable form of movement that remains feasible even in the presence of symptoms. This research applied inferential statistical analysis using Spearman's rank-order correlation to assess the relationships between variables, resulting in a correlation matrix with Spearman's rho values and corresponding p-values. Findings indicate positive effects of regular physical activity in mitigating MS symptoms such as fatigue, mobility difficulties, and cognitive impairments. Beyond physical benefits, exercise contributes to a greater sense of control over the disease and enhances social and emotional well-being.

A specific feature of this study is its focus on individuals living on the Dalmatian coast, where climatic factors—especially elevated temperatures for most of the year—further influence exercise adaptations, particularly due to the common occurrence of heat intolerance in people with MS. Accordingly, the importance of a personalized exercise approach is emphasized, aligned with current recommendations from the National MS Society (USA), which include physical activity guidelines tailored to all levels of functional ability.

Keywords: multiple sclerosis, exercise intervention, Spearman's correlation, recreational sport.

INTRODUCTION

When a person—including a recreational athlete—is diagnosed with a condition such as multiple sclerosis (MS), understanding the role of physical activity in disease management becomes crucial. Studies have shown that regular exercise can positively impact various aspects of life for individuals with MS, including mood enhancement, improved strength, balance, and functional mobility, as well as reduced fatigue (Latimer-Cheung et al., 2013). Although physical inactivity and sedentary behavior are relatively common among people with MS, growing evidence supports the idea that individualized exercise can improve both physical and psychological health and quality of life (Latimer-Cheung et al., 2013; Motl & Pilutti, 2012). Nevertheless, challenges such as fatigue, heat intolerance, and mobility limitations often hinder consistent exercise participation, especially in recreational athletes. These symptoms require specific modifications to exercise routines (Motl & Pilutti, 2012). Consequently, fitness routines must evolve to reflect the fluctuating symptoms of MS in recreational athletes. This approach aligns with current guidelines emphasizing individualized exercise programming to optimize benefits and minimize risks (Dalgas et al., 2019). While recreational athletes may not maintain previous fitness levels, they continue to adapt their routines to incorporate exercise as an integral part of daily life (Androja et al., 2020). Ongoing adaptation and mindful engagement with one's capabilities and limitations are key to successful long-term disease management through physical activity (Miočić & Komšo, 2020). This study addresses the lack of understanding regarding how recreational athletes with MS adapt their training regimens over time in response to evolving symptoms, particularly from the perspective of lived experience (Du et al., 2024). There is a recognized need to explore subjective experiences of exercise among individuals with MS to inform realistic, sustainable, and motivating exercise programs that account for the challenges of this unpredictable disease. The aim of this paper is to explore and present the personal experience of exercise adaptation in recreational athletes living with MS and to compare these insights with current scientific knowledge. The study combines personal narrative and literature review to highlight the importance of a flexible, individualized approach to physical activity in MS. Research questions include: How do recreational athletes with MS perceive and adapt their training over time?, How can these subjective experiences be reconciled with scientific recommendations for physical activity?, What are the most common challenges to maintaining regular training among individuals with MS?

Context and Personal Perspective

For many individuals, physical exercise was an integral part of their identity and daily routine prior to being diagnosed with multiple sclerosis (MS). As long-time recreational athletes, they were accustomed to a dynamic lifestyle that included various forms of physical activity such as hiking, water sports, running, functional training, and occasional participation in amateur competitions. However, the diagnosis of MS introduced a profound shift in how these individuals perceive, experience, and engage in physical activity. The onset of initial symptoms—such as chronic fatigue, heat sensitivity, and intermittent limb weakness—significantly affected their ability to maintain previous levels of physical performance. Initially, many continued with their usual training intensity, often ignoring the changes. However, as Motl and Pilutti (2012) point out, individuals with MS who do not adjust their activity intensity may experience worsening symptoms and further declines in quality of life.

Moving forward, recreational athletes are compelled to adopt a different mindset—transitioning from someone who "pushes physical limits through training" to someone who exercises with the goals of preserving functionality, reducing symptoms, and maintaining mental stability and social inclusion. As such, training becomes perceived less as a means to athletic progression and more as a therapeutic tool. This shift in perspective is supported by existing literature, which recognizes physical activity as an "informal intervention for symptom management, preserving independence, and improving quality of life in individuals with MS" (Latimer-Cheung et al., 2013, p. 1801). This process necessitates acceptance of flexibility in training—adapting the duration, intensity, and type of activity to the body's daily condition (Miočić et al., 2020). According to Rodríguez and colleagues (2021), on days when symptoms are mild, individuals engage in short functional workouts using body weight, whereas during periods of pronounced fatigue, exercise routines consist of light stretching and breathing exercises. This approach aligns with the recommendations of Dalgas et al. (2019), who emphasize the importance of individualized and appropriate physical activity in people with MS. Beyond physical benefits, exercise helps individuals retain a sense of continuity and control—maintaining connection with the "athlete I was before the diagnosis" (Miočić & Komšo, 2020). As Grazioli et al. (2019) suggest, although the athletic identity is altered, it remains present—now redefined as that of a person who consciously engages in exercise as a form of self-care and self-sustenance.

METHODES

This study employed a mixed methods design, integrating qualitative autoethnographic approaches with quantitative descriptive statistics. This combination enabled the integration of the subjective dimension of personal experience with objective patterns of behavior and perception within a broader population of individuals diagnosed with multiple sclerosis (MS) who engage in physical activity.

Qualitative Component. The qualitative portion of the study was based on autoethnography, a research method that blends autobiographical writing with ethnographic analysis (Ellis, Adams, & Bochner, 2011; Sparkes, 2000). Participants—recreational athletes diagnosed with MS—maintained diary entries, retrospective notes, and reflective essays over a six-month period. The collected narrative data covered topics such as training adaptations, emotional responses, and shifts in perceptions of physical activity. The data were analyzed using the thematic analysis method proposed by Braun and Clarke (2006), which allows for the identification of patterns of meaning within qualitative data. Three key themes emerged from the analysis: Redefinition of athletic identity, Flexibility and adaptation of the training process, Psychological significance and function of exercise in managing disease symptoms.

Quantitative Component. The quantitative segment of the research involved descriptive statistical analysis derived from a structured online questionnaire. The study sample included 40 recreational athletes with MS, aged 28 to 62 years ($M = 44.2$; $SD = 8.1$), consisting of 60% women ($n = 24$) and 40% men ($n = 16$). The questionnaire comprised the following thematic sections:Demographic data (age, gender, disease duration), Exercise habits (frequency, duration, type of activity), Perceived exercise intensity (self-assessed), and Self-assessment of the impact of MS symptoms on daily functioning and ability to engage in physical activity.

The goal of the quantitative analysis was to identify patterns in exercise behavior and perception among individuals with MS, and to compare these findings with the results of the qualitative (autoethnographic) analysis, in order to construct a more comprehensive understanding of the experience of physical activity in the context of MS.

For additional scientific rigor, an inferential statistical method was applied—Spearman's rank-order correlation (Field, 2013)—to examine the relationships among four variables: disease duration, exercise frequency, exercise intensity, and the perceived impact of MS symptoms. The resulting data analysis yielded a correlation matrix with Spearman's rho values and associated p-values for significance testing.

RESULTS AND DISCUSSION

The quantitative findings serve to complement the qualitative insights, affirming that the author's personal experiences are not isolated, but rather reflect broader patterns among recreational athletes with multiple sclerosis (MS) who strive to maintain an active lifestyle. Both qualitative and quantitative analyses reveal a complex and dynamic adaptation process in physical activity among individuals with MS, with a particular emphasis on the importance of maintaining a sense of identity and control through movement.

Practical Implications of the Research Findings

The study results suggest several key guidelines for working with recreational athletes diagnosed with MS, especially those with a history of regular training:

- A) Flexibility in Training Program Design Training programs should be dynamic and adaptable to the individual's current physical condition. This involves modifications in intensity, duration, and type of activity according to daily fluctuations in symptoms (Dalgas et al., 2019).

- B) Preservation of Identity Through Movemen. For recreational athletes, exercise is not merely a physical activity, but part of their personal identity. Training should support a sense of continuity with their "athletic self," even if through modified forms of physical activity.

- C) Psychosocial Support Through Exercis. Survey results show that 92.5% of participants report a positive psychological effect of exercise. Incorporating physical activity as a therapeutic tool within multidisciplinary rehabilitation can play a key role in preserving mental health.

- D) Interdisciplinary Collaboratio. Optimal support for individuals with MS involves collaboration among professionals such as physiotherapists, kinesiologists, neurologists, and psychologists, ensuring that physical activity is integrated into holistic health care.

Key Descriptive Statistics 85% of participants (n = 34) reported the need to modify their training regimen after MS diagnosis. 72.5% (n = 29) exercised 2–4 times per week, while only 10% (n = 4) trained more than four times weekly. The most common types of activity reported were: Walking (78%), Stretching (62%), Swimming (38%), Light functional training (35%) and 47.5% identified fatigue as the greatest barrier to regular training, followed by balance and coordination difficulties (25%).

A significant 92.5% (n = 37) of participants stated that engaging in physical activity positively affected their mental health, particularly in relation to stress, anxiety, social connectedness, and perceived control.

Further Interpretation and Thematic Findings Redefinition of Athletic Identity.

4. Autoethnographic reflections revealed a gradual, emotionally demanding shift in identity—from someone who trains to increase fitness and performance to someone who exercises for self-preservation. This transformation is supported by the survey results, where 92.5% reported that exercise contributes to maintaining psychological stability. This aligns with previous research highlighting the mental health benefits of physical activity in individuals with MS (Latimer-Cheung et al., 2013).

5. Adaptation of the Training Process. Descriptive statistics showed that the majority (85%) regularly adjust the form, duration, and intensity of their exercise based on daily symptom variability. As previously noted, the most common activities include walking (78%), stretching (62%), swimming (38%), and functional training (35%). These activities are typically low to moderate in intensity, consistent with current recommendations for people with MS (Dalgas et al., 2019). The author's personal experience further validates the necessity for flexibility, as days with more pronounced symptoms often limit activity to light stretching and breathing exercises.

Table 1. *Most Common Types of Activity Among Recreational Athletes with MS*

Type of Activity	Percentage (%)
Walking	78%
Stretching	62%
Swimming	38%
Functional training	35%

3. Perceived Barriers and the Importance of Adaptation. Fatigue was identified as the main barrier to physical activity by 47.5% of participants, while 25% reported balance-related problems. These findings align with the literature, which identifies fatigue as one of the strongest predictors of reduced physical activity in people with MS (Motl & Pilutti, 2012). Despite these challenges, most participants found ways to maintain some form of physical activity, shifting exercise from a "recreational" practice to a means of **self-care**, as evidenced by the survey results. This redefinition of the role of physical activity in participants' lives highlights the importance of **developing individualized and flexible training programs** that account for the physical, emotional, and identity-related dimensions of living with this chronic condition.

Table 2. *Perceived Main Barriers to Engaging in Physical Activity*

Type of Barrier	Percentage (%)
Fatigue	47.5%
Balance problems	25%
Other barriers	27.5%

Study Limitations, Like any research, this study has certain limitations: **Sample size**: The quantitative analysis is based on a relatively small sample (n = 40), limiting generalizability. **Subjectivity of the autoethnographic approach**: While autoethnography provides rich, in-depth insights, it is inherently subjective and cannot represent all individuals with MS. **Self-reported data**: All quantitative data rely on self-reporting, which may be subject to social desirability bias and inaccurate assessments. **Symptom variability in MS**: Due to the heterogeneous nature of the disease, drawing universal conclusions applicable to all individuals with MS is challenging.

Table 3. *Frequency of Physical Activity in Recreational Athletes with MS*

Exercise Frequency	Percentage (%)
2–4 times per week	72.5%
More than 4 times per week	10%
Less than 2 times per week	17.5%

Correlational Analysis. Spearman's rank correlation analysis was conducted to examine relationships among four variables: duration of illness, frequency of exercise, intensity of exercise, and perceived impact of MS symptoms. The results (Pallant, 2020) show that none of the correlations reached statistical significance (all $p > 0.05$). However, a slight positive relationship was observed between exercise frequency and exercise intensity ($\rho = 0.260$), as well as between exercise frequency and perceived symptom impact ($\rho = 0.265$). Correlations involving illness duration were weak or negligible.

Table 4. Spearman's Correlation Between Key Variables

Variables	ρ (rho)	p-value
Duration of illness – Exercise frequency	–0.017	0.919
Duration of illness – Exercise intensity	0.088	0.593
Duration of illness – Symptom impact	0.116	0.481
Exercise frequency – Exercise intensity	0.260	0.110
Exercise frequency – Symptom impact	0.265	0.103
Exercise intensity – Symptom impact	0.151	0.360

CONCLUSION

This study highlights that, despite the numerous challenges brought on by a diagnosis of multiple sclerosis (MS), physical activity remains a crucial factor in preserving quality of life, personal identity, social inclusion, and psychological stability among recreational athletes. By integrating autoethnographic insight with quantitative data, it was found that individuals with MS rarely abandon exercise altogether. Instead, they redefine and adapt it, using training as a **therapeutic tool**. The findings point to several key needs: A sensitized, multidimensional approach by professionals who understand the specific challenges of living with MS, The development of adaptable training models, offering flexibility according to fluctuating symptoms, Greater awareness of the psychological value of exercise, even when performed in minimal amounts. To deepen the analytical scope of the study, a Spearman's rank-order correlation was conducted, revealing a slight positive association between exercise frequency and intensity ($\rho = 0.26$), and between exercise frequency and perceived symptom impact ($\rho = 0.265$). Ultimately, physical activity emerges as **a** space of resistance against the disease—a domain where the individual retains an active role in their own health, not only through bodily movement but also through the meaning they assign to motion, rhythm, and the discipline of everyday social life. Future research could expand on this work by: Conducting longitudinal studies tracking changes in exercise engagement across different stages of the disease, Comparing distinct subgroups (e.g., previously active vs. inactive individuals with MS), Including larger and more diverse samples, as well as in-depth qualitative interviews to better understand individual adaptation strategies and Exploring the potential of digital tools and online exercise programs for people with MS — particularly in the context of accessibility and self-monitoring of progress.

REFERENCES

16. Androja, L., Miočić, J., Bilić, Ž., & Komšo, M. (2021). Frequency of peripheral nerve injuries in athletes of certain sports clubs in the city of Zadar. *Acta Kinesiologica, 15*(1), 127–132. https://doi.org/10.51371/issn.1840-2976.2021.15.1.1

17. Braun, V., & Clarke, V. (2006). Using thematic analysis in psychology. *Qualitative Research in Psychology, 3*(2), 77–101. https://doi.org/10.1191/1478088706qp063oa

18. Dalgas, U., Langeskov-Christensen, M., Stenager, E., & Riemenschneider, M. (2019). Exercise as medicine in multiple sclerosis—Time for a paradigm shift: Preventive, symptomatic, and disease-modifying aspects and perspectives. *Current Neurology and Neuroscience Reports, 19*(11), 88. https://doi.org/10.1007/s11910-019-1004-7

19. Du, L., Xi, H., Zhang, S., Zhou, Y., Tao, X., Lv, Y., Hou, X., & Yu, L. (2024). Effects of exercise in people with multiple sclerosis: A systematic review and meta-analysis. *Frontiers in Public Health, 12*, Article 1387658. https://doi.org/10.3389/fpubh.2024.1387658

20. Ellis, C., Adams, T. E., & Bochner, A. P. (2011). Autoethnography: An overview. *Forum: Qualitative Social Research, 12*(1), Article 10. https://doi.org/10.17169/fqs-12.1.1589

21. Field, A. (2013). *Discovering statistics using IBM SPSS statistics* (4th ed.). Sage Publications.

22. Grazioli, E., Tranchita, E., Borriello, G., Cerulli, C., Minganti, C., & Parisi, A. (2019). The effects of concurrent resistance and aerobic exercise training on functional status in patients with multiple sclerosis. *Current Sports Medicine Reports, 18*(12), 452–457. https://doi.org/10.1249/JSR.0000000000000661

23. Latimer-Cheung, A. E., Pilutti, L. A., Hicks, A. L., Ginis, K. A. M., Fenuta, A. M., MacKibbon, K. A., & Motl, R. W. (2013). Effects of exercise training on fitness, mobility, fatigue, and health-related quality of life among adults with multiple sclerosis: A systematic review to inform guideline development. *Archives of Physical Medicine and Rehabilitation, 94*(9), 1800–1828.e3. https://doi.org/10.1016/j.apmr.2013.04.020

24. Mitchell, C. H., Brushant, T. M., Shivani, A., Belzberg, A. J., Corrino, J. A., & Fayad, L. M. (2014). MRI of sports-related peripheral nerve injuries. *AJR American Journal of Roentgenology, 203*(5), 1075–1084. https://doi.org/10.2214/AJR.13.11844

25. Miočić, J., & Komšo, M. (2020). Važnost tjelesnog vježbanja za osobe s dijagnosticiranom multiplom sklerozom. *Zbornik Sveučilišta Libertas, 5*(5), 27–34. https://doi.org/10.46672/zsl.5.5.2

26. Miočić, J., Androja, L., & Čular, D. (2020). Understanding the significance of cannabidiols and their possible use in sport. *International Journal of Innovative Science and Research Technology, 5*(7). [ISSN: 2456-2165]

27. Motl, R. W., & Pilutti, L. A. (2012). The benefits of exercise training in multiple sclerosis. *Nature Reviews Neurology, 8*(9), 487–497. https://doi.org/10.1038/nrneurol.2012.136

28. Pallant, J. (2020). *SPSS survival manual: A step-by-step guide to data analysis using IBM SPSS* (7th ed.). McGraw-Hill Education.

29. Rodríguez Fuentes, G., Silveira Pereira, L., Ferradáns Rodríguez, P., & Campo Prieto, P. (2022). Therapeutic effects of the Pilates method in patients with multiple sclerosis: A systematic review. *Journal of Clinical Medicine, 11*(3), 683. https://doi.org/10.3390/jcm11030683

30. Sparkes, A. C. (2000). Autoethnography and narratives of self: Reflections on criteria in action. *Sociology of Sport Journal, 17*(1), 21–43. https://doi.org/10.1123/ssj.17.1.21

Determining the Difference Between the Chronological and Biological Age of Athletes Diagnosed with Trigeminal Neuralgia

original research article

Asst. Prof. PhD. Josip Miočić, Center for Physical Education and Student Sports, University of Zadar. 0000-0002-2508-383X - josip miocic (josip.miocic@szgz.hr)

Milica Komšo, Md. Zadar General Hospital.

Abstract: Trigeminal neuralgia induces severe, often intolerable pain in patients—athletes, in this context—that is frequently resistant to currently available therapeutic options. The International Association for the Study of Pain (IASP) defines trigeminal neuralgia as a sudden, typically unilateral, intense, brief, stabbing, and recurring episode of pain in the distribution of one or more branches of the trigeminal nerve. The condition may be caused by vascular compression of the trigeminal nerve, tumor-related processes, or multiple sclerosis. Compression of the nerve itself leads to demyelination, which results in abnormal depolarization and the generation of ectopic impulses. Triggers for pain may include heat, cold, eating, breathing, tooth brushing, shaving, or incidental contact. Once diagnosed by a specialist, magnetic resonance imaging (MRI) is required to confirm or exclude multiple sclerosis. Tumorous processes may also secondarily lead to trigeminal neuralgia. The first-line pharmacological treatment remains carbamazepine. If pharmacotherapy proves ineffective, more invasive interventions such as microvascular decompression, stereotactic radiosurgery (Gamma Knife), percutaneous balloon microcompression, glycerol rhizolysis, and radiofrequency (RF) ablation may be considered. This study is unique in that its sample comprises athletes diagnosed with trigeminal neuralgia. The primary objective is to examine potential differences between their chronological and biological age by analyzing their metabolic age. The findings aim to support and potentially initiate a novel paradigm or theoretical framework concerning the remodeling of biological aging in athletes suffering from trigeminal neuralgia, particularly in the context of optimizing training processes.

Keywords: trigeminal neuralgia, athletes, chronological age, biological age.

Introduction

Trigeminal neuralgia, also referred to as "tic douloureux," is characterized by extremely sharp, episodic, intense, stabbing facial pain. The pain is localized within the innervation zone of one of the trigeminal nerve branches—most commonly the second or third—and significantly diminishes the patient's quality of life (Dlaka & Vasung, 2007). It is a chronic pain disorder affecting the trigeminal nerve, which transmits sensory information from the face to the brain. To fully grasp the nature of trigeminal neuralgia, one must first understand neuralgia itself, which is defined as episodic irritation of a nerve that produces intense neural pain along a damaged nerve pathway. In cases of trigeminal neuralgia, even mild facial stimuli such as brushing teeth or applying makeup can provoke intense pain or distress.

The pain is typically described as stabbing, occurring in paroxysms at consistent locations and with consistent intensity (Scrivani, Mathews, & Maciewicz, 2005). The trigeminal nerve is one of the most important cranial nerves. According to Merskey and Bogduk (1994), damage to this nerve generally results in severe unilateral facial pain. In modern medicine, due to advances in diagnostic and treatment modalities, trigeminal neuralgia no longer necessarily condemns the patient to a lifetime of suffering. Although not life-threatening, it can severely impair physical functioning and quality of life.

There is currently no objective diagnostic test for trigeminal neuralgia; diagnosis relies entirely on clinical expertise and recognition of its distinct symptoms (Chudy et al., 2012). Patients experience sharp, stabbing pain on the affected side of the face, lasting from seconds to a minute. According to Apfelbaum (2000), the pain can be triggered by light touch, air drafts, or spontaneous neural activity. Attacks may recur at progressively shorter intervals until they become nearly continuous. In some instances, the pain is accompanied by muscle spasms that lead to visible facial tics.

As Chudy and colleagues (2012) explain, trigeminal neuralgia involves a disruption of trigeminal nerve function, often resulting from contact between a blood vessel (artery or vein) and the nerve within the brain. This contact exerts pressure on the nerve, disrupting and damaging its function. Additionally, trigeminal neuralgia can be associated with conditions such as multiple sclerosis, particularly in younger individuals. In such cases, the pain may be bilateral and involve the ophthalmic branch, resulting in sensory disturbances in the forehead region (Fukuda, Ishikawa, & Okumura, 2003).

Initial treatment typically involves pharmacological intervention. For many patients, this is sufficient (Scrivani, Mathews, & Maciewicz, 2005). However, due to variations in individual physiology and disease progression, medications can lose efficacy over time or produce adverse effects. For such cases, modern medicine offers injections or surgical procedures, including microvascular decompression and other techniques, which can effectively manage the disorder (Chudy et al., 2012).

According to Perrudin (2005), sport as a structured physical activity engages both physical and psychological dimensions, with an inherent social component. These characteristics make sport highly relevant to overall health and well-being, encompassing physical, mental, and social domains (Mijolović, 2014). At its core, sport consists of rule-governed physical activity aimed at progress in physical, psychological, and social development (Wikipedia, 2024). Just like the general population, athletes diagnosed with trigeminal neuralgia endure intense pain that interferes with their daily lives and primary sporting activities.

Pathopsychology

According to Tolle, Dukes, and Sadosky (2006), trigeminal neuralgia most commonly occurs in middle-aged and elderly individuals, including athletes. In the literature, it is described as paroxysmal pain of extreme intensity, with burning, stabbing, and tearing characteristics. Merskey and Bogduk (1994) report that it is most often localized within the maxillary and mandibular branches of the trigeminal nerve and, less frequently, the ophthalmic branch. Patients frequently describe it as the most excruciating pain imaginable—akin to electric shocks, lightning strikes, stabbing, tearing, or burning sensations across the face.

To emphasize the severity of this condition, Tomasović (2019) notes that there have unfortunately been documented cases of suicide among patients who could no longer endure the pain. Typically, the pain episodes are brief, lasting only a few seconds to one minute, but their intensity can provoke involuntary facial muscle contractions, including tonic-clonic spasms of the eye and cheek. Following an attack, patients may experience autonomic symptoms such as facial flushing, lacrimation, nasal discharge, or salivation (Dionne, Newton-John, & Zakrzewska, 2009). Despite the frequency of these attacks, patients experience pain-free intervals between episodes.

As previously mentioned, pain can be triggered by minimal facial stimulation, speech, chewing, or exposure to cold air. In severe cases, patients may avoid all movement and contact, including speaking or eating, to prevent triggering pain—

resulting in what is sometimes described as the "mummy face." Due to reduced food intake, patients—particularly athletes—often experience significant weight loss over short periods.

The condition typically begins with alternating periods of pain and remission, complicating the structuring of a consistent training regimen. According to Androja et al. (2021), pain episodes may persist for several months before spontaneously resolving. However, Radoš (2004) observes that over time, painful periods lengthen and pain-free intervals shorten, ultimately leading to a state of continuous pain in all patients. After prolonged disease progression, approximately one-quarter of patients develop sensory deficits in the area innervated by the trigeminal nerve (Radoš, 2004).

Symptomatic trigeminal neuralgia occurs when the nerve is irritated by an underlying pathological condition such as multiple sclerosis, vascular compression, a basilar artery aneurysm, or a pontocerebellar tumor. Numerous studies and authors report that sensory loss on the face and diminished corneal reflexes are characteristic findings. Miočić and Komšo (2020) emphasize that diagnosis is primarily clinical, although magnetic resonance imaging (MRI) in idiopathic cases may reveal dilation of the superior cerebellar artery loop, exerting pressure on the nerve and leading to demyelination. According to Tomasović (2019), in younger patients, trigeminal neuralgia most frequently arises as a consequence of demyelinating lesions or neoplasms.

Sport and Trigeminal Neuralgia

For athletes, physical movement, active engagement, communication, and dynamic social interaction are essential to participating in sports. The coexistence of such a physically demanding lifestyle with a condition as debilitating as trigeminal neuralgia appears paradoxical—yet it occurs. Athletes diagnosed with this disorder face daily battles to maintain functionality and continue their professional activities.

Imagine an individual for whom deep breathing, swallowing, chewing, or even speaking triggers excruciating pain—described as akin to a needle prick or an electric shock. Now, imagine that this individual is a professional athlete. According to Chong et al. (2023), trigeminal neuralgia is widely recognized in both medical and public discourse due to the extreme facial pain it causes. Affecting approximately 12 out of every 100,000 individuals worldwide (Machado, Ogrin, Rosenow, & Henderson, 2021), the condition's rarity makes its presence among elite athletes particularly noteworthy.

Although the identities of affected athletes are generally kept private, an exception can be made in the case of Álvaro Morata, a prominent football player and member of the Spanish national team. Public reports have confirmed that Morata suffers from trigeminal neuralgia (Sport, 2024). His club, Atlético Madrid, has openly expressed concern, highlighting that although the condition is rare, it poses a significant challenge to maintaining a normal lifestyle and consistent football training.

The lead author of this paper, himself a former athlete and now an official in the sports sector, also lives with what he refers to as a "condition" rather than a disease—trigeminal neuralgia. Like others—both athletes and non-athletes—he contends with pain episodes that arise suddenly, last for varying durations over days or weeks, and then subside. This erratic pattern inevitably impacts quality of life, professional obligations, and the ability to participate in either competitive or recreational physical activity. Nevertheless, his experience serves as evidence that coexisting with such a condition, while difficult, is possible.

As previously noted, diagnosing this disorder is far from straightforward, especially in athletes, for whom time-sensitive performance requirements demand rapid medical clarity. There is no definitive diagnostic test; diagnosis depends heavily on patient interviews and thorough clinical and neurological examinations. According to Professor Klepac, diagnostic procedures are primarily aimed at ruling out other conditions that may mimic trigeminal neuralgia. These include vascular compression, tumors, or demyelinating diseases such as multiple sclerosis (Xu & Jackson, 2021).

Timely medical consultation is essential, as chronic pain severely compromises quality of life. In conclusion, trigeminal neuralgia is a neurological condition that causes chronic facial pain due to damage or dysfunction of the trigeminal nerve. It presents significant obstacles for athletes, hindering both their routine training activities and their ability to maintain a full quality of life.

Chronological and Biological Age

According to Vásquez-Alvarez et al. (2021), chronological age is measured in years from an individual's date of birth. A crucial distinction exists between how many years a person has lived—referred to as chronological age—and the overall condition of their body, known as biological age. This difference can help demystify the aging process and support a more holistic and robust approach to health assessment.

As noted by Mišigoj-Duraković et al. (2018), biological or physiological age can be defined as an individual's capacity to adapt to environmental conditions, most commonly expressed through endurance, strength, flexibility, coordination, and work capacity. Both chronological and biological age serve as metrics for understanding aging and the impact of time on the human body. Chronological age quantifies the number of years a person has lived. According to Pisaruk et al. (2021), individuals born in the same year share the same chronological age regardless of how old or young they may appear or feel.

In contrast, biological age varies between individuals and more accurately reflects the diversity in aging processes. Donma and Donma (2020) argue that biological age reveals how a person is aging based on numerous factors and biomarkers. However, no single biomarker or diagnostic test can definitively determine a person's age. Various studies have advanced the theoretical framework in this domain. For instance, Paolisso, Barbieri, Bonafè, and Franceschi (2001) proposed a new paradigm—the theory of aging remodeling. This has been further developed by researchers such as Kusnoputranto et al. (2020) and Pisaruk et al. (2021).

Materials and Methods

The study was conducted in Croatia, where, based on the authors' knowledge and the available literature, a total of 46 athletes from various sports disciplines and competitive levels diagnosed with trigeminal neuralgia (G50.0) were included. Statistical analysis was performed using the Statistica 14.0 software package, with the level of significance set at $p < 0.05$.

Descriptive statistical parameters were calculated, including arithmetic mean (AM), standard deviation (SD), minimum (MIN), and maximum (MAX) values. To determine differences between chronological age and metabolic age among participants, a paired-samples t-test was applied. Furthermore, to examine the relationship between the variables representing the difference between chronological and metabolic age, a correlation analysis using Pearson's correlation coefficient was conducted.

Prior to the measurement of morphological variables, participants completed a questionnaire containing personal data, including their chronological age (CA). The morphological status variables used in the research included body mass, hydration status, fat mass, lean mass, and muscle mass, all measured using the Tanita BC-418 body composition analyzer, which employs bioelectrical impedance analysis. Body height was assessed using an anthropometer.

Based on the results obtained from the morphological measurements, the Tanita device calculated each participant's metabolic age (MA). For the purpose of this study, the difference between chronological age and metabolic age (CA–MA) was subsequently calculated and analyzed.

Results

An athlete's chronological age may serve as one indicator of their physical conditioning relative to other athletes. In contrast, metabolic age reflects the athlete's basal metabolic rate in comparison with peers. In other words, if an athlete's chronological age aligns with their metabolic age, this suggests that the athlete's physiological status is consistent with that of the broader athletic population within the same age range.

Table 1: *Descriptive Statistical Indicators of the Applied Variables (N – number of participants, AM – arithmetic mean, SD – standard deviation, MIN – minimum value, MAX – maximum value)*

	N	AS	SD	MIN	MAX
KD	46	66.08	5.56	51.00	78.00
MD	46	52.45	8.41	38.00	72.'00
KD-MD	46	12.89	8.69	-14-00	17.00
ST	46	132.10	23.04	90	166.00
DT	46	76.62	10.04	51.00	95.00
FS	46	72.40	10.01	51.00	94.00

Legend: KD – chronological age, **MD** – metabolic age, **KD-MD** – difference between chronological and metabolic age, **ST** – systolic pressure, **DT** – diastolic pressure, **FS** – heart rate

The research findings emphasize the fact that elevated heart rate is a strong predictor of cardiovascular mortality—more commonly observed in men (Palatini et al., 1999)—and that it is essential to monitor heart rate regularly, both at rest and during physical activity in athletes.

Table 2. Results of the Paired-Samples t-Test (Differences Between Chronological and Metabolic Age)

	AS	SD	N	t	df	p
KD	64.07	5.65	46	9.44	41.00	0.00
MD	51.40	8.79				

Legend: KD – chronological age, **MD** – metabolic age

The results of the paired-samples t-test (Table 2) confirmed the hypothesis regarding the statistical significance of differences between the chronological and metabolic age of participants engaged in recreational exercise programs ($p = 0.00$). Additionally, the t-test results confirmed the significance of differences between chronological and metabolic age among participants involved in professional sports programs ($p = 0.00$). These significant differences highlight the fact that metabolic age is a much stronger predictor of cardiovascular risk than chronological age (Elguezabal-Rodelo et al., 2021).

Table 3. Results of the Correlation Analysis Between Cardiac Functions (Systolic and Diastolic Blood Pressure and Heart Rate) and the Difference Between Chronological and Metabolic Age

	KD-MD	FS	DT	ST
KD-MD	1.00	-	-	-
FS	-0.14	1.00	-	-
DT	-0.51	0.16	1.00	-
ST	-0.19	0.006	0.65	1.00

Legend: KD-MD – difference between chronological and metabolic age, **ST** – systolic pressure, **DT** – diastolic pressure, **FS** – heart rate

Within this study, the only statistically significant correlation was observed between the difference in chronological and metabolic age and diastolic blood pressure ($r = -0.51$). A higher basal metabolic rate was associated with lower diastolic pressure. Although this outcome is logically coherent, it contrasts with several previous findings

(Seghieri et al., 2008). It is important to emphasize that the study sample predominantly consisted of male participants, most of whom were classified as non-obese.

Conclusion

The conducted research established a significant difference between the chronological and metabolic age of athletes diagnosed with trigeminal neuralgia. Furthermore, the findings confirmed the paradigm that there is a meaningful correlation between heart rate and the difference between chronological and metabolic age among the examined athletes. In addition, a significant association was observed between diastolic blood pressure and the difference between chronological and metabolic age in the same population.

These results support the premise that professional athletes affected by trigeminal neuralgia—a condition that causes intense and often debilitating facial pain—may still exhibit a lower metabolic age despite the limitations imposed by their condition. Moreover, participants with a greater discrepancy between chronological and metabolic age also showed lower diastolic blood pressure values, regardless of the influence of trigeminal neuralgia.

The findings contribute valuable insight into the role of biological and chronological age in the context of athletic training among individuals with trigeminal neuralgia. Importantly, the study underscores the need for continued research to further explore this topic and potentially influence how differences between chronological and biological age are assessed in athletes suffering from this neurological condition.

References

Apfelbaum, R. I. (2000). Neurovascular decompression: The procedure of choice? *Clinical Neurosurgery, 46*, 473–498.

Androja, L., Miočić, J., Bilić, Ž., & Komšo, M. (2021). Frequency of peripheral nerve injuries in athletes of certain sports clubs in the city of Zadar. *Acta Kinesiologica, 15*(1), 127–132. https://doi.org/10.51371/issn.1840-2976.2021.15.1.1

Chong, M. S., Bahra, A., & Zakrzewska, J. M. (2023). Guidelines for the management of trigeminal neuralgia. *Cleveland Clinic Journal of Medicine, 90*(6), 355–362.* https://doi.org/10.3949/ccjm.90a.22098*

Chudy, D., Dlaka, D., Almahariq, F., Romić, D., Marković, D., & Grahovac, G. (n.d.). Mikrovaskularna dekompresija u supinacijskom položaju za liječenje neuralgije trigeminusa. *Medicina.*

Dlaka, D. (2007). *Prognostički čimbenici i čimbenici ishoda liječenja radiokirurgijom gama nožem bolesnika oboljelih od refraktorne idiopatske neuralgije trigeminusa* [Master's thesis, Hrvatski institut za istraživanje mozga]. Zagreb.

Dionne, R., Newton-John, T., & Zakrzewska, J. M. (2009). Overall management of facial pain. In J. M. Zakrzewska (Ed.), *Orofacial pain* (pp. 53–68). Oxford University Press.

Donma, O., & Donma, M. M. (2020). Assessment of obesity parameters in terms of metabolic age above and below chronological age in adults. *International Journal of Medical and Health Sciences, 14*(2), 65–68.

Elguezabal-Rodelo, R., Ochoa-Précoma, R., Vazquez-Marroquin, G., Porchia, L. M., Montes-Arana, I., Torres-Rasgado, E., Méndez-Fernández, E., Pérez-Fuentes, R., & Gonzalez-Mejia, M. E. (2021). Metabolic age correlates better than chronological age with waist-to-height ratio, a cardiovascular risk index. *Medicina Clínica (Barcelona), 157*(9), 409–417. https://doi.org/10.1016/j.medcli.2020.07.026

Fukuda, H., Ishikawa, M., & Okumura, R. (2003). Demonstration of neurovascular compression in trigeminal neuralgia and hemifacial spasm with magnetic resonance imaging: Comparison with surgical findings in 60 consecutive cases. *Surgical Neurology, 59*, 93–100. https://doi.org/10.1016/S0090-3019(02)01014-5

Lopez, B. C., Hamlyn, P. J., & Zakrzewska, J. M. (2022). Stereotactic radiosurgery for primary trigeminal neuralgia: State of the evidence. *Acta Clinica Croatica, 61*(Suppl. 2), 100–106.

Machado, A., Ogrin, M., Rosenow, J. M., & Henderson, J. M. (2007). A 12-month prospective study of Gasserian ganglion stimulation for trigeminal neuropathic pain. *Stereotactic and Functional Neurosurgery, 85*, 216–224.

Merskey, H., & Bogduk, N. (1994). *Classification of chronic pain: Descriptions of chronic pain syndromes and definitions of pain terms* (2nd ed.). IASP Press.

Miočić, J., & Komšo, M. (2020). Važnost tjelesnog vježbanja za osobe s dijagnosticiranom multiplom sklerozom. *Zbornik Sveučilišta Libertas, 5*(5), 27–34. https://doi.org/10.46672/zsl.5.5.2

Perrudin, F. (2005). *Civilizacije svijeta.* Naša djeca.

Pisaruk, A., Shatilo, V., Shchehlova, I., Naskalova, S., & Mechova, L. (2021). Model of human metabolic age. *Problems of Endocrine Pathology, 77*(3), 71–75.

Radoš, M. (2004). Trigeminal neuralgia and recommendations for future reports. *Journal of Neurology, Neurosurgery & Psychiatry, 75*, 1019–1024.

Scrivani, S. J., Mathews, E. S., & Maciewicz, R. J. (2005). Trigeminal neuralgia. *Oral Surgery, Oral Medicine, Oral Pathology, Oral Radiology, and Endodontology, 100*(5), 527–533. https://doi.org/10.1016/j.tripleo.2005.05.044

Tolle, T., Dukes, E., & Sadosky, A. (2006). Patient burden of trigeminal neuralgia: Results from a cross-sectional survey of health state impairment and treatment patterns in six European countries. *Pain Practice, 6*, 153–160.

Tomasović, S. (2019). Nuralgije kranijalnih živaca. *Medicus, 28*(1), 71–75.

Vásquez-Alvarez, S., Bustamante-Villagomez, S. K., Vazquez-Marroquin, G., Porchia, L. M., Pérez-Fuentes, R., Torres-Rasgado, E., & Gonzalez-Mejia, M. (2021). Metabolic age, an index based on basal metabolic rate, can predict individuals that are high risk of developing metabolic syndrome. *High Blood Pressure & Cardiovascular Prevention, 28*(3), 263–270.

Xu, R., Xie, M. E., & Jackson, C. M. (2021). Trigeminal neuralgia: Current approaches and emerging interventions. *Journal of Pain Research, 14*, 3437–3463. https://doi.org/10.2147/JPR.S314372

www.ingramcontent.com/pod-product-compliance
Lightning Source LLC
LaVergne TN
LVHW051130210926
848482LV00001B/48
* 9 7 9 8 8 9 9 6 6 4 8 9 2 *